Bala

Gliclazide Mucoadhesive Microcapsu

Bala Vishnu Priya Mukkala
T.E.G.K. Murthy

Gliclazide Mucoadhesive Microcapsules:Impact of Process Variables

Benefits of Gliclazide mucoadhesive microcapsules

LAP LAMBERT Academic Publishing

Impressum/Imprint (nur für Deutschland/only for Germany)
Bibliografische Information der Deutschen Nationalbibliothek: Die Deutsche Nationalbibliothek verzeichnet diese Publikation in der Deutschen Nationalbibliografie; detaillierte bibliografische Daten sind im Internet über http://dnb.d-nb.de abrufbar.
Alle in diesem Buch genannten Marken und Produktnamen unterliegen warenzeichen-, marken- oder patentrechtlichem Schutz bzw. sind Warenzeichen oder eingetragene Warenzeichen der jeweiligen Inhaber. Die Wiedergabe von Marken, Produktnamen, Gebrauchsnamen, Handelsnamen, Warenbezeichnungen u.s.w. in diesem Werk berechtigt auch ohne besondere Kennzeichnung nicht zu der Annahme, dass solche Namen im Sinne der Warenzeichen- und Markenschutzgesetzgebung als frei zu betrachten wären und daher von jedermann benutzt werden dürften.

Coverbild: www.ingimage.com

Verlag: LAP LAMBERT Academic Publishing GmbH & Co. KG
Heinrich-Böcking-Str. 6-8, 66121 Saarbrücken, Deutschland
Telefon +49 681 3720-310, Telefax +49 681 3720-3109
Email: info@lap-publishing.com

Approved by: Submitted to Jawaharlal Nehru Technological University, Kakinada, 2011

Herstellung in Deutschland (siehe letzte Seite)
ISBN: 978-3-659-15798-1

Imprint (only for USA, GB)
Bibliographic information published by the Deutsche Nationalbibliothek: The Deutsche Nationalbibliothek lists this publication in the Deutsche Nationalbibliografie; detailed bibliographic data are available in the Internet at http://dnb.d-nb.de.
Any brand names and product names mentioned in this book are subject to trademark, brand or patent protection and are trademarks or registered trademarks of their respective holders. The use of brand names, product names, common names, trade names, product descriptions etc. even without a particular marking in this works is in no way to be construed to mean that such names may be regarded as unrestricted in respect of trademark and brand protection legislation and could thus be used by anyone.

Cover image: www.ingimage.com

Publisher: LAP LAMBERT Academic Publishing GmbH & Co. KG
Heinrich-Böcking-Str. 6-8, 66121 Saarbrücken, Germany
Phone +49 681 3720-310, Fax +49 681 3720-3109
Email: info@lap-publishing.com

Printed in the U.S.A.
Printed in the U.K. by (see last page)
ISBN: 978-3-659-15798-1

Process Variables and their Impact on Performance of Gliclazide Mucoadhesive Microcapsules

Benefits of Gliclazide mucoadhesive microcapsules

Edited by

Bala Vishnu Priya Mukkala, M.Pharm.

and

Dr. T.E.G.K. Murthy, M.Pharm., Ph.D.

RESUME:

Author:

Bala Vishnu Priya Mukkala, awarded M.Pharmacy degree with specialization in Pharmaceutics from Bapatla College of Pharmacy affiliated to Jawaharlal Nehru Technological University, Kakinada.

Co-author:

Dr. T.E.Gopala Krishna Murthy presently assuming the office of Principal, Bapatla College of Pharmacy, Bapatla was awarded M.Pharmacy Degree from BIT, Ranchi and Ph.D from JNTU, Hyderabad. Published more than 150 research papers and guided 10 Ph.D students, conferred with meritorious teacher award from JNTUK in 2010 and fellowship from Association of Pharmacy & Biotechnology.

ACKNOWLEDGMENTS:

The authors are grateful to Aurobindo Pharmaceuticals, Hyderabad and Management of Bapatla College of Pharmacy, Bapatla for providing necessary requirements.

Table of Contents

1. INTRODUCTION...……...…....7-22
   a. Scope and objectives
   b. Advantages and disadvantages of controlled drug delivery systems
   c. Characteristics of drugs suitable and un-suitable for controlled release
   d. Approaches for oral controlled release drug delivery systems
   e. Microcapsules
   f. Mucoadhesive microcapsules
   g. Theories of bioadhesion
   h. Mechanism of mucoadhesion
   i. Factors affecting mucoadhesion
   j. Advantages & disadvantages of mucoadhesive systems
   k. Preparation of mucoadhesive microcapsules
   l. Evaluation of mucoadhesive microcapsules

2. EXPERIMENTAL INVESTIGATION..............................…...24-71
   a. Estimation of gliclazide
   b. Infrared spectroscopic studies
   c. Preparation of gliclazide microcapsules
   d. Characterization of gliclazide microcapsules
   e. Pharmaco-dynamic studies on rabbits

3. SUMMARY, CONCLUSION and RECOMMENDATIONS.....73-75

4. REFERENCES...…...77-81

INTRODUCTION

SCOPE AND OBJECTIVES

Gliclazide is an oral hypoglycemic second generation sulfonyl urea drug which is useful for a long-term treatment of non-insulin dependent diabetes mellitus (NIDDM). For an oral hypoglycemic drug, rapid absorption from the gastrointestinal tract is required for an effective pharmacological activity. The absorption rate of gliclazide from the gastrointestinal tract is slow and varied among the subjects. The slow absorption has been suggested to be due to either poor dissolution of gliclazide owing to its hydrophobic nature or poor permeability of the drug across the GI membrane. Incorporation of gliclazide in controlled release dosage forms may regulate its absorption from the gastrointestinal tract and overcome the variability problems. The modified-release preparation demonstrates very high bioavailability and allows reduction in the effective dose .It reduces the glycosylated haemoglobin (HbA1C) levels and minimizes the side effects with less risk of hypoglycemia.

Microencapsulation is a useful method to prolong the drug release from dosage forms and reducing adverse effects. Microparticles are defined as spherical polymeric particles. These microparticles constitute an important part of these novel drug delivery systems, by virtue of their small size and efficient carrier characteristics. However, the success of these novel microparticles is limited due to their short residence time at the site of absorption. If these drug delivery systems provide an intimate contact with the absorbing membranes then they will become an effective drug delivery. It can be achieved by coupling bioadhesion characteristics to microparticles and developing novel delivery systems referred to as "bioadhesive microparticles". Bioadhesive microparticles include microspheres and microcapsules (having a core of the drug) of 1– 1000 μm in diameter and consisting either entirely of a bioadhesive polymer or having an outer coating of it. Bioadhesive microparticles have advantages such as efficient absorption and enhanced bioavailability of drugs owing to their high surface to volume ratio, a

7

much more intimate contact with the mucus layer, and specific targeting of drugs to the absorption site. The main objective of this investigation is partial curing of sodium alginate to retain its muco adhesiveness property and allowing the retarded release due to the formation of calcium alginate. Exposure of sodium alginate to calcium chloride reagent leads to the formation of calcium alginate which is hydrophobic and non muco adhesive. Thus gliclazide is allowed to deposited with the combination of sodium alginate (muco adhesive polymer) and calcium alginate (non muco adhesive layer) The extent and rate of drug release from microcapsules is affected by various formulation variables and different processing conditions such as stirring speed, stirring time, volume of curing reagent, concentration of curing reagent and curing time So the effect of these parameters was studied and results are reported here.

The main objectives of the present work are as follows

1. To design, develop and characterization of mucoadhesive microcapsules for gliclazide.

2. To prepare the gliclazide microcapsules by employing ionic gelation technique.

3. To study the influence of stirring speed on drug loading and in vitro drug release rate of gliclazide microcapsules

4. To study the influence of curing time on drug loading and in vitro drug release rate of gliclazide microcapsules.

5. To study the influence of stirring time on drug loading and in vitro drug release rate of gliclazide microcapsules.

6. To study the influence of volume of curing reagent on drug loading and in vitro drug release rate of gliclazide microcapsules.

8

7. To study the influence of concentration of curing reagent on drug loading and in vitro drug release rate of gliclazide microcapsules.

8. To evaluate the kinetics and mechanism of drug release from the microcapsules.

9. To conduct the compatibility studies between drug and polymer by FT-IR studies

10. To characterize the optimized formulation of gliclazide microcapsules.

11. To compare the optimized formulation of gliclazide microcapsules with marketed formulations.

12. To carry out pharmacodynamic studies on rabbit

Controlled release (CR) technology has rapidly emerged over the last three decades as a new interdisciplinary science that offers novel approaches to the delivery of one or more bioactive agents continuously in a predetermined pattern for a fixed period of time either systemically or to a specified target organ. The ability to control the drug release kinetics is such that the drug delivery for days and years can be achieved[1].

By achieving a predictable and reproducible bioactive agent release rate for an extended period of time, CR formulations can achieve optimum therapeutic responses, prolonged efficacy, and also decreases the toxicity.

The primary objectives of controlled release drug delivery systems are to ensure safety and to improve efficacy of drugs as well as patient compliance. This is achieved by better control of plasma drug levels and less frequent dosing[2]

1.1 Advantages and disadvantages of controlled drug delivery systems:

The advantages of controlled drug delivery systems are as follows

1. Decreased incidence and or intensity of adverse effects and toxicity
2. Better drug utilization
3. Controlled rate and site of release
4. More uniform blood concentrations
5. Improved patient compliance
6. Reduced dosing frequency
7. More consistent and prolonged therapeutic effect
8. A greater selectivity of pharmacological activity

Disadvantages of controlled drug delivery systems:

1. Increased variability among dosage units
2. Stability problems
3. Toxicity due to dose dumping
4. Increased cost
5. More rapid development of tolerance
6. Need for additional patient education and counseling

1.2. Characteristics of drugs suitable and un-suitable for controlled release:

The drugs which are satisfying the following requirements are the suitable candidates for oral controlled drug delivery.

1. Exhibit moderate rates of absorption and excretion
2. Uniform absorption throughout the GI tract
3. Administered in relatively small doses eg. L - DOPA
4. Possess a good margin of safety
5. For the treatment of chronic therapy eg: anti anxiety drugs-alprazolam, diazepam

Characteristics of drugs un-suitable for controlled release:

1. Not effectively absorbed in the lower intestine (riboflavin)
2. Absorbed and excreted rapidly, short biologic half-lives,< 1hr (Pencillin G, furosemide)
3. Long biological half-lives > 12 hr (diazepam, phenytoin)
4. Large doses required, 1g (sulfonamides)
5. Drugs with low therapeutic index (Phenobarbital, digoxin)

11

6. Precise dosage titrated to individuals required (anti coagulants, cardiac glycosides)

7. No clear advantage for sustained release formulation (griseofulvin)

Controlled release drug delivery systems have been designed for oral, parenteral, implantation and transdermal routes. Oral route is the most convenient and most common mode of administration of controlled release systems.

The efficiency of oral drug delivery depends on various factors such as type of delivery system, the disease being treated, the patient, the length of the therapy and the properties of the drug. Most of the oral controlled drug delivery systems (OCDDS) relay on diffusion, dissolution, or combination of both mechanisms. The physico-chemical properties of the drug such as crystal nature, solubility, partition coefficient, intrinsic dissolution; etc are known to influence the efficacy. Dosage form characteristics are controlled and optimized based on the physic-chemical properties of the drug, relevant GI environmental factors. Other factors need to be considered are disease state, the patient compliance & length of therapy.

1.3 Approaches for oral controlled release drug delivery systems[3]:

The design and fabrication of oral controlled release systems are classified based on the mechanism of drug release as

1. Dissolution controlled release
2. Diffusion controlled release
3. Diffusion and dissolution controlled release
4. Ion-exchange resins

5. pH- dependent formulations

6. Osmotically controlled release

7. Altered density formulations/ buoyant systems

Controlled release systems for oral use includes systems in the form of

- Coated pellets
- Matrix tablets
- **Microcapsules**
- Poorly soluble drug complexes
- Ion exchange resin complexes
- Osmotic pumps etc.,

These systems are designed to release drug over an extended period of time, either in a continuous manner (Sustained release) or as a series of pulses (timed release). Among the various approaches, microspheres and microcapsules have gained good acceptance as a process to achieve controlled release.

1.4. Microcapsules

Microencapsulation is a well designed controlled drug delivery system to overcome the problems of conventional therapy and enhance the therapeutic efficacy of a given drug. To obtain maximum therapeutic efficacy, it becomes necessary to deliver the agent to the target tissue in the optimal amount in the right period of time there by causing little toxicity and minimal side effects. Among the various approaches, microspheres are best one to deliver the drug in a controlled manner. Microencapsulation is the process of application of relatively thin coatings to small particles of solids and or droplets of liquids or dispersions. The capsule shell can be designed to release their contents at a specific set of conditions. Both biodegradable and non-biodegradable materials have been investigated for the preparation of microspheres. The term microcapsule is defined as a spherical particle with size ranging from 50nm to 2mm, containing a core substance[4].

There are many reasons to encapsulate the drugs and related chemicals include[5]:

- To mask the bitter taste of the drugs like paracetamol, Nitrofurantoin etc.
- To reduce gastric and other GI irritations. E.g. Aspirin, which causes gastric bleeding.
- To stabilize the drugs those are sensitive to oxygen, moisture or light. e.g. Vitamin A Palmitate
- To reduce the hygroscopic properties of the core material e.g. Ranitidine HCI Amoxycillin, Clavulanic acid, vitamins and cloxacilin
- To reduce the odour and volatility. e.g. Methyl salisylate
- To separate the incompatible substances
- To improve the handling and storage of a liquid. Liquids can be converted in to a pseudo-solid. e.g.Eprazinone.
- To alter the site of absorption

Types of microcapsules:
- Biodegradable microcapsules
- Non-biodegradable microcapsules
- Magnetic microcapsules
- **Mucoadhesive microcapsules**
- Gastroretentive microcapsules (Floating microcapsules)

14

However, the success of these microcapsules is limited due to their short residence time at the site of absorption. It would, therefore be advantageous to have means for providing an intimate contact of the drug delivery system with the absorbing membranes. This can be achieved by coupling the mucoadhesive characteristics to microcapsules and developing **mucoadhesive microcapsules**[6].

1.5. Mucoadhesive microcapsules

The term bioadhesion refers to any bond formed between two biological surfaces or a bond between a biological and synthetic surface. In case of bioadhesive drug delivery systems, the term bioadhesion is used to describe adhesion between polymers either synthetic or natural and soft tissues (GI mucosa). Mucoadhesive drug delivery systems utilizes the property of bioadhesion of certain polymers which become adhesive on hydration and hence can be used for targeting a drug to a particular region of the body for extended periods of time.

Mucoadhesive microcapsules include microparticles and microcapsules of 1-1000 mm in diameter and consisting either entirely of a mucoadhesive polymer or having an outer coating of it respectively. Mucoadhesive microcapsules offer efficient absorption and enhanced bioavailability owing to their high surface to volume ratio, which provides intimate contact with the mucus membrane and specific targeting of drugs to the absorption site.

Mucoadhesive microcapsules can be designed to adhere to any mucosal tissue including those found in eye, nasal cavity, urinary and gastrointestinal tract, thus offering the possibilities of localized as well as systemic controlled release of drugs. Application of mucoadhesive microcapsules to the mucosal tissues of ocular cavity, gastric and colonic epithelium is used for administration of drugs for localized action. Prolonged release of drugs and a reduction in frequency of

15

drug administration to the ocular cavity can highly improve the patient compliance. The latter advantage can also be obtained for drugs administered intra-nasally due to the reduction in mucociliary clearance of drugs adhering to nasal mucosa[7].

1.5.1 Theories of bioadhesion[8]:

Many theories have been proposed to explain the forces responsible for bioadhesion. They are

- Electronic theory,
- Adsorption theory,
- Diffusion theory,
- Wetting theory and
- Fracture theory.

These theories have been proposed to explain the mechanism of interactions between the polymers and glycoproteins, though each provides only a partial explanation, that is the formation of the close contact between the mucoadhesive polymer and the biological tissue, which is mediated by the suitably moist surface of the mucosa and swelling of the adhesive.

1.5.2. Characteristics of Bioadhesive polymer[8, 9]:

It has been stated that at least one of the following characteristics are required to obtain adhesion. Each of these characteristics favors the formation of bonds that are either chemical or mechanical in nature.

a. Sufficient quantities of hydrogen bonding chemical groups

b. Anionic surface

c.   High molecular weight

d.   High chain flexibility and

e.   Surface tension that will induce spreading into mucous layer

1.5.3. Mechanism of mucoadhesion[8-10]:

The mechanism involved in the formation of bioadhesive bonds in between the polymer hydrogels and soft tissues has been described in three steps.

a. **Step 1:** The wetting and swelling step occurs when the polymer spreads over the surface of the biological substrate or mucosal membrane in order to develop an intimate contact with the substrate. Bioadhesives are able to adhere to or bond with biological tissues by the help of the surface tension and forces that exist at the site of the adsorption or contact. Swelling of polymers occurs because the components within the polymers have an affinity for water.

b. **Step 2:** The surface of the mucosal membranes are composed of high molecular weight polymers known as glycoproteins. In step 2 of the bioadhesive bond formation, the bioadhesive polymer chains and the mucosal polymer chains intermingle and entangle to form semi-permeable adhesive bonds. The strength of these bonds depends on the degree of penetration between the two polymer groups. In order to form strong adhesive bonds, one polymer group must be soluble in the other and both polymer types must be of similar chemical structure.

c. **Step 3:** Formation of weak chemical bonds between entangled chains. The types of bonding formed between the chains include primary bonds such as covalent bonds and weaker secondary interactions such as van der Waals interactions and hydrogen bonds. Both primary and secondary bonds are exploited in the manufacture of bio-adhesive formulations in which strong adhesions between polymers are formed.

1.5.4. Polymers used for mucoadhesive microcapsules[11, 12]:

Mucoadhesive delivery systems are being explored for the localization of the active agents to a particular location/ site. Polymers have played an important role in the designing such systems so as to increase the residence time of the active agent at the desired location. The properties of mucoadhesive microcapsules, e.g. surface characteristics, force of mucoadhesion, release pattern of the drug and clearance are influenced by the type of the polymers used to prepare them.

Characteristics of an ideal mucoadhesive polymer[13-16]:

- Display a high level of bio- and mucoadhesion
- Readily synthesized in bulk
- Soluble in aqueous solutions (physiologic pH range)
- Non toxic to the epithelium
- Degradation products should be non toxic and not absorbable in GI tract
- Promote the improvement of barrier function
- High molecular weight (up to 100 or more), high viscosity and spatial conformation
- Flexibility of polymer which promotes the interpenetration of the polymer with in mucous network
- Optimum degree of cross linking, hydration and optimum concentration of the polymer

- Charge on the mucoadhesive polymer, the mucoadhesive strength can be attributed as anion>cation>nonionic.
- The polymer must not decompose on storage or during the shelf life of the dosage form.

1.5.5. Factors affecting mucoadhesion [11, 17, 18]:

Mucoadhesion is a property of both the bioadhesive polmer and the medium in which it is placed. The characterstics of the mucoadhesive polymer and mucosa, as well as other factors which can affect the strength and duration of the strength of mucoadhesive interaction are summarized below:

➢ **Polymer related factors:**
- Molecular weight,
- Concentration of polymer
- Polymer chain flexibility
- Ability to form hydrogen bond
- Extent of swelling of polymer

➢ **Physical factors**
- pH at polymer substrate interface
- Applied strength
- Initial contact time
- Moistening
- Presence of metal ions

➢ **Physiological factors**
- Mucin turnover rate
- Diseased state
- Tissue movement

1.5.6. Advantages & disadvantages of mucoadhesive systems[7, 19]:

The advantages offered by these systems are furnished below.

- Prolongs the residence time of the dosage form at the site of absorption. Due to an increased residence time it enhances absorption and hence the therapeutic efficacy of the drug
- Readily localized in the region applied to improve and enhance the bioavailability of drugs. E.g: testosterone and its esters, vasopressin, dopamine, insulin and gentamycin
- Excellent accessibility
- These dosage forms facilitate intimate contact of the formulation with underlying absorption surface, which allows modification of tissue permeability for absorption of macromolecules. E.g: peptides and proteins, sodium glycocholate, sodium taurocholate and L- lysophoaphotidyl choline.
- Rapid absorption because of enormous blood supply and good blood flow rates
- Increase in drug bioavailability due to avoidance of first pass metabolism
- Drug is protected from degradation in the acidic environment in the GIT
- Improved patient compliance- ease of drug administration
- Faster onset of action is achieved due to mucosal surface

Disadvantages of mucoadhesive systems:

Medications administered orally do not enter the blood stream immediately after passage through the buccal mucosa. They have to be swallowed and then have passed through a portion of the GIT before being absorbed. So the action is not very rapid in the GIT as compared when the drug is administered through buccal route.

1.5.7. PREPARATION OF MUCOADHESIVE MICROCAPSULES[7, 20]:

The mucoadhesive microcapsules can be prepared by employing any of the following techniques

- ➤ Ionic gelation and emulsification ionic gelation

- ➤ Solvent evaporation

- ➤ Coacervation phase separation

- ➤ Hot melt microencapsulation

- ➤ Solvent removal method

- ➤ Spray drying and spray congealing

- ➤ Phase inversion microencapsulation

- ➤ Pan coating

1.5.8. EVALUATION OF MUCOADHESIVE MICROCAPSULES[21-23]:

The Mucoadhesive microcapsules are evaluated for the following parameters.

2. Size and shape

3. Entrapment efficiency

4. Drug content or % drug loading

5. In vitro drug release studies

6. Micromeretic properties

7. Moisture content

8. Surface accumulation

9. Wall thickness

10. Swelling index

11. Erosion

12. Degree of cross linking

13. In vitro wash-off test

14. Adhesive strength

15. Tensile stress measurement

16. Fracture strength

17. Deformation to failure

18. Work of adhesion

19. Shear stress measurement

20. Adhesion number

21. Falling liquid film method

22. Everted sac technique

23. Measurement of residence time

24. GI transit using radio opaque microspheres

25. Gamma scintigraphy technique

EXPERIMENTAL INVESTIGATION

Materials and Methods:

The following materials were used in the present research work.

Gliclazide was procured from Aurobindo pharmaceuticals, Hyderabad as a gift sample. Sodium alginate and calcium chloride were obtained from SD Fine chemicals, Mumbai. Hydrochloric acid, sodium acetate, glacial acetic acid, potassium dihydrogen phosphate, sodium hydroxide, and acetonitrile AR purchased from Qualigens fine chemicals, Mumbai were used in this investigation. UV- Visible spectrophotometer (Shimadzu, UV- 1700), magnetic stirrer (Remi Motors, Model No RO123R, Mumbai), mechanical stirrer (Remi Motors Pvt. Limited, Mumbai), 8 stage dissolution test apparatus (Shimadzu, TDT 08L, Mumbai), and hot air oven (Thermo Labs), Mumbai were used in this investigation.

Estimation of gliclazide:

The following analytical methods are reported for the estimation of Gliclazide:

1. Spectrophotometry[24,25]
2. Gas liquid chromatography (GLC)[26,27]
3. Thin layer chromatography (TLC)[28]
4. High performance liquid chromatography (HPLC)[29,30]
5. Reverse phase High performance liquid chromatography (RP-HPLC) [31,32]
6. Non-aqueous titration (Titrimetry)[33]
7. Radioimmunoassay[34]

In this investigation UV-Visible spectrophotometric method was used for the estimation of Gliclazide.

Determination of the λ_{max}:

Accurately weighed amount of Gliclazide (25mg) was dissolved in 10 ml of acetonitrile and further diluted with phosphate buffer pH 7.4 up to 25ml. Then the solution was scanned for maximum absorbance in UV double beam spectrophotometer (Shimadzu, UV-1700) in the range from 200 to 400 nm using phosphate buffer pH 7.4 as blank. The λ_{max} of the drug was found to be 227 nm.

Construction of calibration curve for gliclazide:

Preparation of standard solution of gliclazide: Accurately weighed amount of gliclazide (25 mg) was transferred to a 25 ml volumetric flask, dissolved in acetonitrile and the volume was adjusted up to the mark.

Procedure:

The standard solution of gliclazide was subsequently diluted with phosphate buffer pH 7.4 to obtain a series of dilutions containing 2- 10 µg of gliclazide per ml of solution. The absorbance of these solutions was measured in Shimadzu double beam UV spectrophotometer at 227 nm using phosphate buffer pH 7.4 as blank. The absorbance values were plotted against concentration of gliclazide as shown in Figure 1. The method obeyed Beer's law in the concentration range of 2-10 µg/ ml.

Figure 1: Calibration curve of gliclazide in phosphate buffer pH 7.4

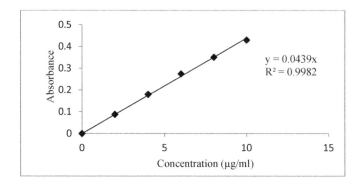

Infrared spectroscopic studies:

Fourier- Transformed Infrared (FT-IR) spectra were obtained on Brucker FT-IR system. The scanning range was 400-4000 cm^{-1}. Drug compatibility studies were performed using FT-IR studies. The IR spectra of the gliclazide, alginate and gliclazide microcapsules are showed in Figure 2-4.

Figure 2: IR spectrum of gliclazide

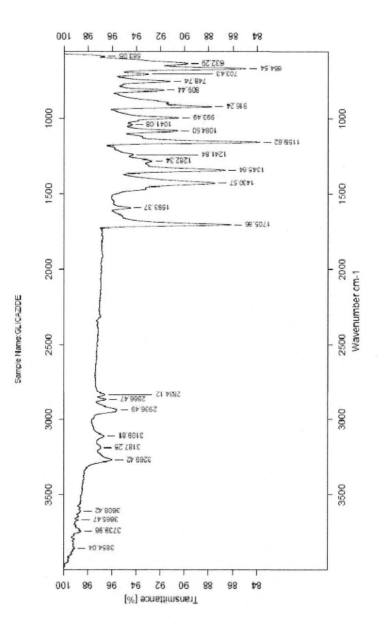

Figure 3: IR spectra of calcium alginate placebo beads / dummy microcapsules

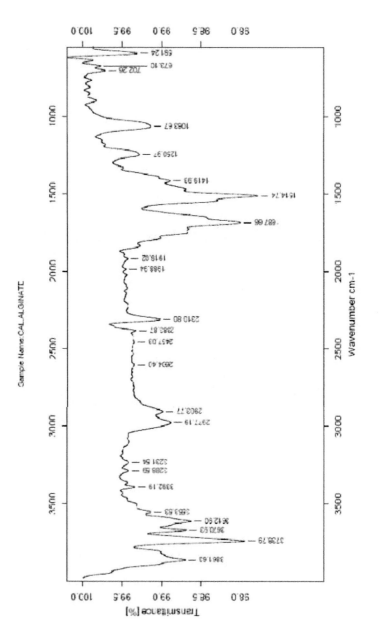

Figure 4: IR spectra of gliclazide microcapsules

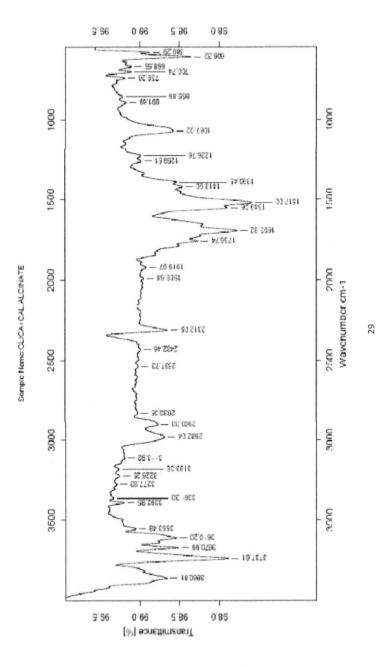

The spectra's of both gliclazide and gliclazide microcapsules were compared and results concluded that there was no interaction observed. C=O streching was observed in case of gliclazide and its microcapsules at 1705.86 cm^{-1} and 1693.82 cm^{-1} respectively. 2° N-H streching was observed in case of gliclazide and its microcapsules at 3269.42 cm^{-1} and 3392.85 cm^{-1} respectively. N-H bending (vibration) was observed in case of gliclazide and its microcapsules at 1593.37 cm^{-1} and 1549.26 cm^{-1} respectively.

Preparation of gliclazide microcapsules[135]:

The gliclazide loaded calcium alginate beads were prepared by employing ionic gelation with and without subjecting to mechanical stirring. The accurately weighed gliclazide (300mg) was dispersed in 10ml of sodium alginate solution (0.6%w/v) and agitated thoroughly on magnetic stirrer to form a viscous homogenous dispersion. Then the dispersion was dropped through the 20mm stainless steel needle into the 150 ml of 0.1M calcium chloride solution, stirred up to 30 min, allowed to retain in calcium chloride solution for curing up to12-72 hrs. The composition and the conditions observed for the preparation of the microcapsules is showed in Table 1.The microcapsules were then separated by decantation, washed three times with deionized water and dried at room temperature for 24hrs.

Initially microcapsules of Gliclazide were formulated by transferring the 0.6% w/v sodium alginate dispersion containing 0.3g of Gliclazide in to 150 ml of 0.1M calcium chloride solution and allowed to stand for 72 hrs. The curing time may influence the entrapment efficiency due to the possible leaching of drug from the

30

microcapsules if they are allowed to retain in the curing reagent even after the completion of curing. If the microcapsules are separated from the curing reagent before completion of curing then the release rate will be less due to improper deposition of calcium alginate as the sodium alginate may not completely converted to calcium alginate. So, to study the effect of curing time on entrapment efficiency and drug release rate, the fraction of microcapsules were collected from the beaker at regular intervals of 12 hrs duration.

Table 1: Composition of microcapsules formulated without stirring and observing different curing times

Formulation	Curing time (hr)	Stirring speed (rpm)	Stirring time (min)	Volume of curing reagent (ml)	Concentration of cross linking agent(M)
F_1	12	0	--	150	0.1
F_2	24	0	--	150	0.1
F_3	36	0	--	150	0.1
F_4	48	0	--	150	0.1
F_5	60	0	--	150	0.1
F_6	72	0	--	150	0.1

The microcapsules were subjected for estimation of drug content and microencapsulation efficiency by employing following procedures.

Drug content[36, 37]:

Microcapsules containing equivalent to 30mg of gliclazide were weighed and crushed to fine powder in a mortar. The drug was extracted with 5 ml of acetonitrile. It was filtered, suitably diluted with phosphate buffer pH 7.4. The drug content was determined from the absorbance measured at 227nm.

Microencapsulation efficiency was calculated using the following formula:

$$\text{Microenapsulation efficiency} = \frac{\text{Estimated drug content}}{\text{Theoretical drug content}} \times 100$$

In vitro drug release study[38]:

Microcapsules containing equivalent to 30 mg of gliclazide were subjected to *In vitro* drug release studies. Release of gliclazide from the beads was studied in phosphate buffer (pH 7.4) using a USP dissolution test apparatus with a rotating basket operated at 100 ± 2 rpm and temperature was maintained at $37\pm$ 1°C. Then at regular intervals of time (30 minutes), 5ml of samples were collected and same volume was replenished with fresh dissolution medium. The withdrawn samples were filtered through what man filter paper (no.41), suitably diluted and analyzed spectrophotometrically at a λ_{max} of 227 using Shimadzu UV-1700 double beam spectrophotometer. The dissolution studies were conducted in triplicate.

The entrapment efficiency observed from these microcapsules collected at different curing times is showed in Table 2. The microencapsulation efficiency is not influenced by the curing time up to 48 hrs later the efficiency was drastically decreased.

Table 2: Entrapment efficiency of gliclazide microcapsules formulated by employing calcium chloride as curing reagent and allowing for curing with different time intervals

Curing time (h)	Drug content (mg)		Encapsulation efficiency (%)
	Theoretical	Practical	
12 (F_1)	30	29.416	98.052
24 (F_2)	30	28.839	96.131
36 (F_3)	30	26.536	88.452
48 (F_4)	30	25.384	84.613
60 (F_5)	30	26.305	87.685
72 (F_6)	30	16.400	54.666

The drug release data observed from these microcapsules is showed in Figure 5. The drug release followed zero order kinetics, as the graph drawn in between amount of drug release vs. time was found to be linear (Figure 6). The n value was found to be nearer to one from peppas plots (Figure7). The drug release from the microcapsules was influenced by curing time. Reduction in release rate was noticed with increased curing time. These studies thus demonstrated the influence of curing time on entrapment efficiency and drug release rate. Optimum curing time is required for better entrapment efficiency and drug release rate. The microcapsules prepared by observing a curing time of 24 hrs yielded an entrapment efficiency of 96.131and the drug release was extended up to 7.5 hrs. The entrapment efficiency was less and higher release rates were noticed from the microcapsules prepared by maintaining the curing time exceeding 24hrs. It may be due to possible leaching of drug from the microcapsules (low entrapment efficiency) and the incidence of higher hydration, subsequent swelling and associated pore formation may favor the release rate of drug (high release rate). The microcapsules formulated by observing a curing time of less than 24 hrs showed good entrapment efficiency and high release rate (Table 3). It may be due to the possible incomplete conversion of sodium alginate to calcium alginate and inadequate deposition of calcium alginate over the Gliclazide. So a curing time of 24 hrs was recommended and selected for further studies.

Figure 5: Comparative in vitro drug release profiles of gliclazide microcapsules formulated by employing calcium chloride as curing reagent and allowing for curing with different time intervals

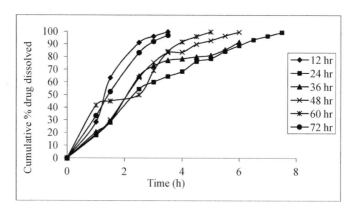

Figure 6: Zero order plots of gliclazide microcapsules formulated by employing calcium chloride as curing reagent and allowing for curing with different time intervals

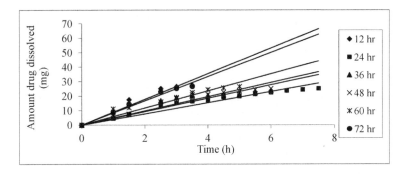

Figure 7: Peppas plots of gliclazide microcapsules formulated by employing calcium chloride as curing reagent and allowing for curing with different time intervals

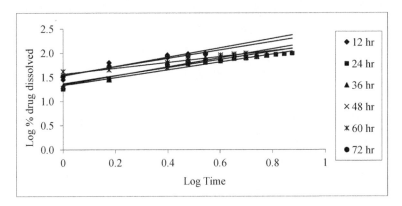

Table 3: In vitro drug release kinetics of gliclazide microcapsules formulated by employing calcium chloride as curing reagent and allowing for curing at different time intervals

Curing time (h)	Correlation coefficient				Release kinetics			Exponential coefficient (n)
	Zero order	First order	Higuchi	Peppas	K mg/h	T_{50} (h)	T_{90} (h)	
12 (F_1)	0.9584	0.8972	0.9555	0.9576	9.9686	1.5	2.7	0.8306
24 (F_2)	0.9526	0.8998	0.9767	0.9820	4.5732	3.3	5.9	0.7363
36 (F_3)	0.9310	0.9800	0.9549	0.9760	5.3642	2.8	5.0	0.8900
48 (F_4)	0.9581	0.9116	0.9562	0.9838	5.8199	2.6	4.6	0.9427
60 (F_5)	0.9556	0.8396	0.9714	0.9465	6.6303	2.3	4.1	0.6052
72 (F_6)	0.9864	0.9510	0.9716	0.9911	9.1259	1.6	3.0	0.8677

In the next step, Gliclazide microcapsules were formulated by transferring the 0.6% w/v sodium alginate dispersion containing 0.3g of Gliclazide in to 150 ml of 0.1M calcium chloride solution which was maintained at 400 rpm and stirring was continued for 30 minutes. Then it was allowed to stand for 72 hrs. To study the effect of curing time on entrapment efficiency and drug release rate, the fraction of microcapsules were collected from the beaker at regular intervals (12 hrs). The composition and the conditions observed for the preparation of the microcapsules is showed in Table 4. The drug content, micro encapsulation efficiency and *in vitro* drug release studies were conducted as described earlier.

Table 4: Composition of microcapsules formulated by maintaining constant stirring and observing different curing times

Formulation	Curing time (hr)	Stirring speed (rpm)	Stirring time (min)	Volume of curing reagent (ml)	Concentration of cross linking agent(M)
F_7	12	400	30	150	0.1
F_8	24	400	30	150	0.1
F_9	36	400	30	150	0.1
F_{10}	48	400	30	150	0.1
F_{11}	60	400	30	150	0.1
F_{12}	72	400	30	150	0.1

The entrapment efficiency observed from these microcapsules is showed in Table 5. The microencapsulation efficiency is not influenced by the curing time up to 48 hrs later the efficiency was drastically decreased.

Table 5:   Entrapment efficiency of gliclazide microcapsules formulated by maintaining an initial stirring of 400 rpm for 30 min and allowing for curing at different time intervals

Curing time (h)	Drug content (mg)		Encapsulation efficiency (%)
	Theoretical	Practical	
12 (F_7)	30	24.002	80.006
24 (F_8)	30	17.552	58.506
36 (F_9)	30	19.894	63.113
48 (F_{10})	30	21.813	72.711
60 (F_{11})	30	16.745	55.818
72 (F_{12})	30	15.433	51.442

The drug release data observed from these microcapsules is showed in Figure 8. The drug release followed zero order kinetics as the graph drawn in between amount of drug release vs. time was found to be linear (Figure 9). The exponential coefficient (n) value of peppas equation was found to be nearer to one (Figure 10). The drug release rate was decreased with increased curing time up to 48hrs. Optimum curing time was required for high entrapment efficiency and drug release rate. In this study the microcapsules formulated by maintaining a curing time of 48hrs yielded an entrapment efficiency of 72.71and the drug release was extended up to 11 hrs. The higher entrapment efficiency and drug release was noticed from the microcapsules formulated by observing curing times less than 48 hrs. Low entrapment efficiency and higher drug release rates was noticed with the microcapsules prepared by maintaining the curing times more than 48hrs (Table 6).

It may be due to variations in extent of calcium alginate deposition. So, a curing time of 48 hrs was selected for further studies.

Figure 8: Comparative in vitro drug release profiles of gliclazide microcapsules formulated by maintaining an initial stirring of 400 rpm for 30 min and allowing for curing at different time intervals

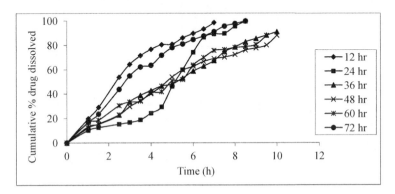

Figure 9: Zero order plots of gliclazide microcapsules formulated by maintaining an initial stirring of 400 rpm for 30 min and allowing for curing at different time intervals

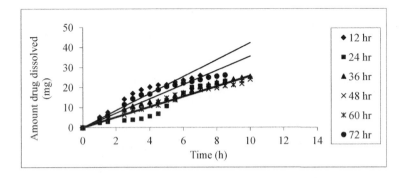

Figure 10: Peppas plots of gliclazide microcapsules formulated by maintaining an initial stirring of 400 rpm for 30 min and allowing for curing at different time intervals

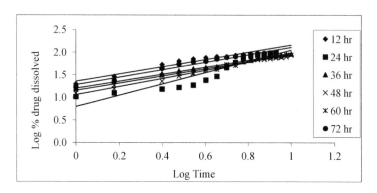

Table 6: In vitro drug release kinetics of gliclazide microcapsules formulated by maintaining an initial stirring of 400 rpm for 30 min and allowing for curing at different time intervals

Curing	Correlation coefficient				Release kinetics			Exponential
time (h)	Zero order	First order	Higuchi	Peppas	K mg/h	T_{50} (h)	T_{90} (h)	coefficient (n)
12 (F_7)	0.9488	0.9282	0.9705	0.9854	4.8560	3.1	5.6	0.7721
24 (F_8)	0.9414	0.7697	0.8007	0.9418	3.3061	4.5	8.2	1.2627
36 (F_9)	0.9805	0.9514	0.9640	0.9916	3.024	5.0	8.9	0.7244
48 (F_{10})	0.9847	0.9750	0.9507	0.9949	2.8002	5.4	9.6	0.8761
60 (F_{11})	0.9822	0.9631	0.9489	0.9740	2.9497	5.1	9.2	0.6901
72 (F_{12})	0.9598	0.8608	0.9729	0.9906	4.0872	3.7	6.6	0.8201

The microcapsules formulated with and without stirring technique were subjected to comparative dissolution studies and the comparative drug release profiles are showed in Figure 11. The results showed a slow drug release from the microcapsules formulated with stirring technique. It may be due to the formation of spherical shaped and smaller size microcapsules. The chance of aggregation tendency is more in case of microcapsules formulated without stirring which may also influence the release rate. The stirring may also allows an efficient contact of dispersion of sodium alginate with the curing reagent and thus allows the formation of calcium alginate. The statistical interpretation of the release rate constant obtained from this two methods indicated a significant difference among the techniques ($p<0.0001$).

Figure 11: Comparative in vitro drug release profiles of gliclazide microcapsules formulated with and without initial stirring

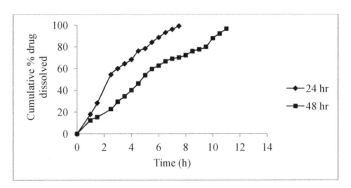

As the stirring was found to influence the encapsulation efficiency and drug release rate from the initial experiments, so microcapsules were formulated by maintaining different intensities (200, 400, 600 and 800 rpm) of agitation while transferring the polymer dispersion in to the curing reagent to study the influence of stirring speeds as shown in Table 7. The drug content, micro encapsulation efficiency and *in vitro* drug release studies were conducted on these microcapsules.

Table 7: Composition of microcapsules formulated with different agitation speeds.

Formulation	Curing time (hr)	Stirring speed (rpm)	Stirring time (min)	Volume of curing reagent (ml)	Concentration of cross linking agent(M)
F_{13}	48	200	30	150	0.1
F_{10}	48	400	30	150	0.1
F_{14}	48	600	30	150	0.1
F_{15}	48	800	30	150	0.1

The encapsulation efficiency of the prepared microcapsules is showed in Table 8. The microencapsulation efficiency was not affected by stirring speed up to 400 rpm and then low entrapment efficiency was noticed.

Table 8: Entrapment efficiency of gliclazide microcapsules formulated with different initial agitation speeds.

Stirring speed (rpm)	Drug content (mg)		Encapsulation efficiency (%)
	Theoretical	Practical	
200 (F_{13})	30	22.277	74.256
400 (F_{10})	30	21.813	72.711
600 (F_{14})	30	17.905	59.682
800 (F_{15})	30	16.540	55.132

The drug release data observed from these microcapsules is showed in Figure 12. The drug release followed zero order kinetics (Figure 13). The n values from peppas plots were found to be nearer to the one (Figure 14). Low drug release rates were observed from the microcapsules formulated by employing the stirring speed of 400 rpm and then release rate was increased with the rpm. It may be due to vortex formation at high agitation rates which was resulted in improper shape of the microcapsules and hence influenced the both encapsulation efficiency and drug release rate (Table 9). It may be due to the improper contact with the curing reagent and also chances of getting aggregating tendency are more with low speed and hence the size and shape of the microcapsules may be altered. Optimum agitation rate is necessary for better entrapment efficiency and drug release rate. The microcapsules formulated by employing stirring speed of 400 rpm yielded an entrapment efficiency of 72.71% and the drug release was extended up to 11 hrs. Hence 400 rpm was selected as an optimum stirring speed for further studies.

Figure 12: Comparative in vitro drug release profiles of gliclazide microcapsules formulated with different initial agitation speeds.

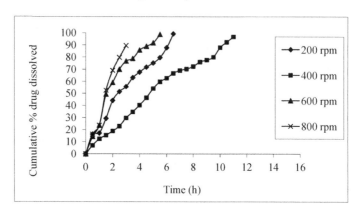

Figure 13: Zero order plots of gliclazide microcapsules formulated with initial agitation speeds.

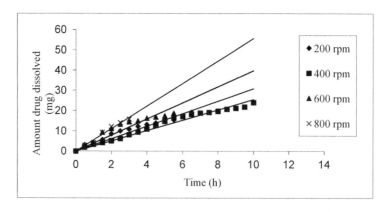

Figure 14: Peppas plots of gliclazide microcapsules formulated with different initial agitation speeds.

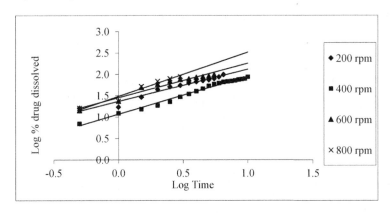

Table 9: In vitro drug release kinetics of gliclazide microcapsules formulated with different initial agitation speeds.

Stirring speed (rpm)	Correlation coefficient				Release kinetics			Exponential coefficient (n)
	Zero order	First order	Higuchi	Peppas	K mg/h	T_{50} (h)	T_{90} (h)	
200 (F_{13})	0.9696	0.0.7973	0.9683	0.9802	4.7675	3.1	5.7	0.7541
400 (F_{10})	0.9847	0.9750	0.9507	0.9949	2.8002	5.4	9.6	0.8761
600 (F_{14})	0.9283	0.9244	0.9742	0.9728	6.2853	2.4	4.3	0.8072
800 (F_{15})	0.9892	0.9594	0.9313	0.9789	9.4504	1.6	2.9	1.0363

As the stirring speed was found to influence the entrapment efficiency and drug release rate, so microcapsules were formulated by maintaining 400rpm of agitation; however the stirring was continued for different time periods (15, 30, 45 and 60 min) after the addition of dispersion in to calcium chloride solution to study the effect of stirring time as shown in Table 10. The microcapsules were evaluated for drug content, micro encapsulation efficiency and *in vitro* drug release studies.

Table 10: Composition of microcapsules formulated with constant stirring speed and various stirring times

Formulation	Curing time (hr)	Stirring speed (rpm)	Stirring time (min)	Volume of curing reagent (ml)	Concentration of cross linking agent(M)
F_{16}	48	400	15	150	0.1
F_{10}	48	400	30	150	0.1
F_{17}	48	400	45	150	0.1
F_{18}	48	400	60	150	0.1

The microencapsulation efficiency from the formulated microcapsules was showed in Table 11. The microencapsulation efficiency was not affected by the stirring time.

Table 11: Entrapment efficiency observed from gliclazide microcapsules formulated by employing various stirring times and constant speed of 400 rpm.

Stirring	Drug content (mg)		Encapsulation
time (min)	Theoretical	Practical	efficiency (%)
15 (F_{16})	30	26.996	89.988
30 (F_{10})	30	21.813	72.711
45 (F_{17})	30	21.880	72.933
60 (F_{18})	30	21.467	71.556

The drug release data observed from these microcapsules is showed in Figure 15. The drug release followed zero order kinetics (Figure 16). The n values from Peppas plots were found to be nearer to the one (Figure 17). Reduction in drug release rate was observed with increased stirring time. The higher drug release was noticed from the microcapsules prepared by maintaining 15 minutes stirring time. Microcapsules formulated with 60 min stirring time yielded an entrapment efficiency of 71.556 and drug release was extended up to 12 hrs (Table 12). Optimum stirring time is required for better entrapment and drug release. So, 60 min stirring time was selected as an optimum stirring time for further studies.

Figure 15: Comparative in vitro drug release profiles of gliclazide microcapsules formulated by employing various stirring times and maintaining 400 rpm

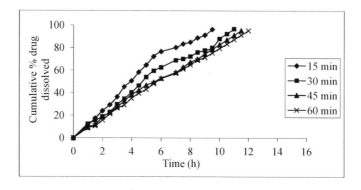

Figure 16: Zero order plots of gliclazide microcapsules formulated by employing various stirring times and maintaining 400 rpm.

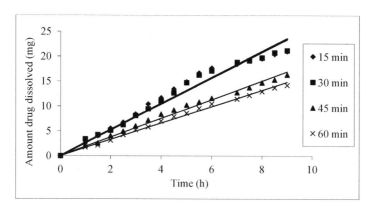

Figure 17: Peppas plots of gliclazide microcapsules formulated by employing various stirring times and maintaining 400 rpm.

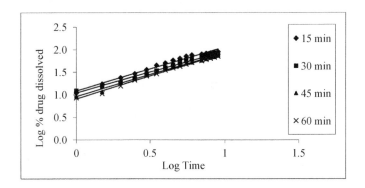

Table 12: In vitro drug release kinetics of gliclazide microcapsules formulated by employing various stirring times and maintaining 400 rpm.

Stirring time (min)	Correlation coefficient				Release kinetics			Exponential coefficient (n)
	Zero order	First order	Higuchi	Peppas	K mg/h	T_{50} (h)	T_{90} (h)	
15 (F_{16})	0.9797	0.9735	0.9412	0.9916	3.4134	4.4	7.9	0.9765
30 (F_{10})	0.9847	0.9750	0.9507	0.9949	2.8002	5.4	9.6	0.8761
45 (F_{17})	0.9949	0.9852	0.9360	0.9959	2.5785	5.8	10.5	0.9715
60 (F_{18})	0.9645	0.8641	0.8670	0.9544	2.4836	6.4	11.5	0.7605

To study the influence of curing reagent solution volume (0.1M Calcium chloride) on efficiency of microcapsules , the microcapsules were formulated by employing different volumes (100, 150 and 200 ml) of the curing reagent (0.1 M $CaCl_2$ solution) and corresponding conditions are shown in Table 13. The drug content, micro encapsulation efficiency and *in vitro* drug release studies were conducted by following the procedures described earlier.

Table 13: Composition of microcapsules formulated with different volumes of curing reagent.

Formulation	Curing time (hr)	Stirring speed (rpm)	Stirring time (min)	Volume of curing reagent (ml)	Concentration of cross linking agent(M)
F_{19}	48	400	60	100	0.1
F_{18}	48	400	60	150	0.1
F_{20}	48	400	60	200	0.1

The entrapment efficiency observed from the formulated microcapsules is showed in Table 14. The entrapment efficiency was found to be increased with increase in the volume of calcium chloride up to 150 ml and then entrapment efficiency decreased with increased volumes of curing reagent solution.

Table 14: Entrapment efficiency of gliclazide microcapsules formulated by employing different volumes of curing reagent

Volume of curing reagent (ml)	Drug content (mg)		Encapsulation efficiency (%)
	Theoretical	Practical	
100 (F_{19})	30	20.817	69.389
150 (F_{18})	30	21.467	71.556
200 (F_{20})	30	19.625	65.417

The drug release data observed from these microcapsules is showed in Figure 18. The drug release followed zero order kinetics (Figure 19). The n values from Peppas plots were found to be nearer to the one (Figure 20). The reduction in entrapment efficiency may due to leaching of the drug in larger volumes of the curing solution. The microcapsules formulated by employing 150 ml of curing reagent solution showed good entrapment efficiency (71.556) and drug release was extended up to12hr (Table 15). Hence 150 ml of curing reagent was selected for further studies.

Figure 18: Comparative in vitro drug release profiles of gliclazide microcapsules formulated by employing curing reagent ((0.1M CaCl$_2$) with varied volumes

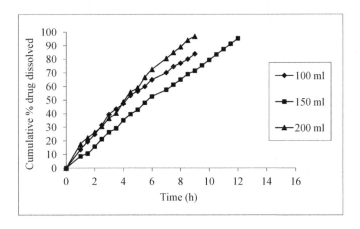

Figure 19: Zero order plots of gliclazide microcapsules formulated by employing curing reagent (0.1M CaCl$_2$) with varied volumes

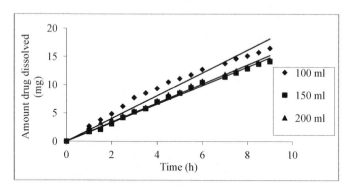

Figure 20: Peppas plots of gliclazide microcapsules formulated by employing curing reagent ((0.1M CaCl$_2$) with varied volumes

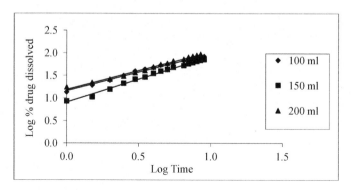

Table 15: In vitro drug release kinetics of gliclazide microcapsules formulated by employing curing reagent ((0.1M $CaCl_2$) with varied volumes

Volume of curing reagent (ml)	Correlation coefficient				Release kinetics			Exponential coefficient (n)
	Zero order	First order	Higuchi	Peppas	K mg/h	T_{50} (h)	T_{90} (h)	
100 (F_{19})	0.9681	0.9662	0.9731	0.99250	2.8780	5.2	9.4	0.7454
150 (F_{18})	0.9645	0.8641	0.8670	0.9544	2.4836	6.4	11.5	0.7605
200 (F_{20})	0.9862	0.8480	0.9540	0.9833	3.340	4.5	8.1	0.7349

The drug release rate from the microcapsules may also influenced by the concentration of curing reagent employed in the preparation of microcapsules. In this investigation, the coating material is formed due to the reaction existing between the polymer and the concentration of curing reagent. So the microcapsules were formulated by employing the various concentrations (0.05, 0.08, 0.1, 0.12 and 0.15M) of curing reagent by maintaining the remaining process variables constant and corresponding composition of microcapsules is shown in Table 16. The drug content, micro encapsulation efficiency and *in vitro* drug release studies were conducted as discussed earlier.

Table 16: Composition of microcapsules formulated with various concentrations of curing reagent.

Formulation	Curing time (hr)	Stirring speed (rpm)	Stirring time (min)	Volume of curing reagent (ml)	Concentration of cross linking agent(M)
F_{21}	48	400	60	150	0.05
F_{22}	48	400	60	150	0.08
F_{18}	48	400	60	150	0.1
F_{23}	48	400	60	150	0.12
F_{24}	48	400	60	150	0.15

The entrapment efficiency observed from the formulated microcapsules is showed in Table 17. The microencapsulation efficiency was dependent on the concentration of the curing reagent and entrapment efficiency was found to be better from the microcapsules formulated with 0.08-0.12M of calcium chloride solution.

Table 17: Encapsulation efficiency of gliclazide microcapsules formulated with various concentrations of curing reagent

Concentration of curing reagent (M)	Drug content (mg)		Encapsulation efficiency (%)
	Theoretical	Practical	
0.05 (F_{21})	30	17.39	57.967
0.08 (F_{22})	30	21.950	73.165
0.1 (F_{18})	30	21.467	71.556
0.12 (F_{23})	30	21.398	71.325
0.15 (F_{24})	30	15.47	51.567

The drug release data observed from these microcapsules is showed in Figure 21. The drug release followed zero order kinetics (Figure 22). The n values from the peppas plots were found to be nearer to the one (Figure 23). Higher drug release rates were noticed from the microcapsules formulated by employing the calcium chloride solution above and below 0.1M concentration (Table 18 and Figure 24). 0.1M concentration was shown good entrapment efficiency 71.556 and drug release was extended up to12hr. So, 0.1M concentration of calcium chloride was selected as optimum concentration for better entrapment efficiency and drug release.

Figure 21: Comparative in vitro drug release profiles of gliclazide microcapsules formulated with various concentrations of curing reagent

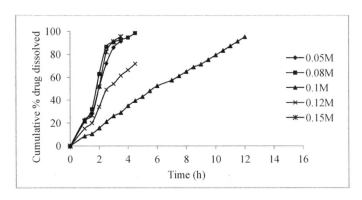

Figure 22: Zero order plots of gliclazide microcapsules formulated with various concentrations of curing reagent

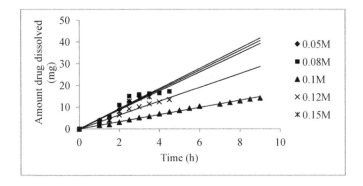

Figure 23: Peppas plots of gliclazide microcapsules formulated with various concentrations of curing reagent

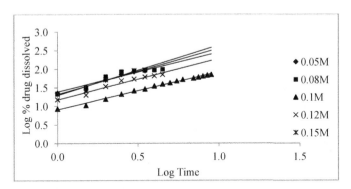

Table 18: In vitro drug release kinetics of gliclazide microcapsules formulated with various concentrations of curing reagent

Concentration of curing reagent (M)	Correlation coefficient				Release kinetics			Exponential coefficient (n)
	Zero order	First order	Higuchi	Peppas	K mg/h	T_{50} (h)	T_{90} (h)	
0.05 (F_{21})	0.9877	0.9574	0.9458	0.9710	9.897	1.5	2.7	0.8618
0.08 (F_{22})	0.9528	0.9483	0.9258	0.9719	7.7450	1.9	3.5	1.0207
0.1 (F_{18})	0.9645	0.8641	0.8670	0.9544	2.4836	6.4	11.5	0.7605
0.12 (F_{23})	0.9900	0.9831	0.9283	0.9825	5.0909	2.9	5.3	0.9661
0.15 (F_{24})	0.9801	0.9430	0.9297	0.9643	10.484	1.4	2.6	0.9413

Figure 24: Relationship between the concentration of curing reagent and release rate constant

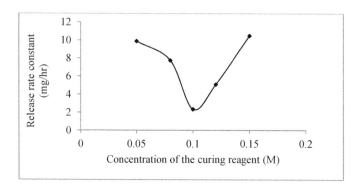

The preliminary investigations were found that the encapsulation efficiency and drug release rate was affected by various formulation factors and processing conditions such as curing time, agitation rate, stirring time, volume of curing reagent and concentration of curing reagent. The composition of the gliclazide microcapsules was optimized and it was found to be the dispersion containing 0.6%w/v sodium alginate, 0.3gm of gliclazide and by employing 150ml of 0.1M calcium chloride as curing reagent. The optimized process variables are 400 rpm agitation for 60 minutes during initial stirring of polymer dispersion with curing reagent solution and maintenance of 48 hr curing time.

Characterization of gliclazide microcapsules:

1. **Rheological properties[39]:**

   Optimized formulation of gliclazide microcapsules was subjected to the determination of following rheological properties:

   a). Bulk density & Tapped density:

   Bulk density and tapped density were measured by using 10 ml graduated cylinder. The previously weighed sample was placed in a cylinder and its initial volume recorded and then subjected to tapping mechanically for 100 times, the corresponding tapped volume was noted down. Bulk density and tapped density were calculated from the following formulae:

   $$\text{Bulk density} = \frac{\text{Mass of microspheres}}{\text{Bulk volume}}$$

   $$\text{Tapped density} = \frac{\text{Mass of microspheres}}{\text{Tapped volume}}$$

   b). Carr's index:

   Carr's index or compressibility index (CI) value of microcapsules was computed with the following equation:

   $$CI\ (\%) = \left|\frac{\rho t - \rho b}{\rho t}\right| \times 100$$

   Where

   ρt - Tapped density

   ρb - Bulk density

c). Hausner's ratio:

Hausner's ratio of the microcapsules was determined by comparing the tapped density to the bulk density using the equation:

$$HR = \frac{\rho t}{\rho b}$$

Where

ρt - Tapped density

ρb - Bulk density

2. Moisture content[40]:

Known quantity of microcapsules was placed in a hot air oven which was maintained at 60°C. At regular time intervals, the microcapsules were withdrawn from the oven and reweighed until the constant weight was attained (equilibrium moisture content). The % moisture content and % loss on drying was calculated with the following formulae:

$$\% \text{ Moisture content} = \frac{\text{Initial weight} - \text{Final weight}}{\text{Final weight}} \times 100$$

$$\% \text{ Loss on drying} = \frac{\text{Initial weight} - \text{Final weight}}{\text{Initial weight}} \times 100$$

3. Physical appearance:

The physical appearance of the microcapsules was observed from the photomicrographs collected from the computer attached trinocular microscope.

4. Swelling index[41]:

The known amount of microcapsules was transferred into a Petri plate containing 25ml of phosphate buffer pH 7.4. At regular intervals of time, the microcapsules were collected and blotted to remove the excess water and reweighed. The swelling index (SI) was measured with following formulae:

$$\text{Swelling index (\%)} = \frac{\text{Final weight} - \text{Initial weight}}{\text{Initial weight}} \times 100$$

5. Erosion study[41]:

The previously weighed microcapsules (W_0) were kept in Petri plate containing 25ml of phosphate buffer pH 7.4. At regular intervals of time, the microcapsules were collected and blotted to remove the excess water and dried in a hot air oven maintained at 50 °C. The weight of the resulting microcapsules was noted as We. The percentage of erosion (E %) was calculated with the following formulae:

$$\text{Erosion (\%)} = \frac{W_0 - W_e}{W_0} \times 100$$

Where

W_0= Initial weight of microspheres

We= weight of eroded microcapsules

6. Wall thickness[42]:

Wall thickness of microcapsules was determined by the method of Luu et al using the equation:

$$h = \frac{\bar{r} \, (1-p) \, d_1}{3[pd_2 + (1-p)d_1 \,]}$$

Where

  h -wall thickness,

$\bar{r}$ -arithmetic mean radius of the coat material,

d_1 -density of the core material

d_2 - density of the coat material

p- Proportion of the medicament in the microcapsules

The true density of the core and coat material was determined using specific gravity bottle. Weight of empty specific gravity bottle was noted as W1 and then the specific gravity bottle was filled with water and its weight was noted as W_2. The solid material (core/coat material) was weighed (500mg), transferred to a specific gravity bottle and then filled with the water. The weight of the bottle after liquid displacement was noted as W_3. The true density of the coating material was determined with the dummy microcapsules (without drug) prepared by employing the procedure described earlier (section 4.4 page 54) without the use of drug. The true density of core and coat material was calculated by the following formula:

$$\text{True density} = \frac{\text{Weight of the solid taken}}{[\,(W2 - W1) + \text{weight of the solid} - (W3)\,]}$$

7. *In vitro* **wash-off test for microcapsules**[43,44]:

The mucoadhesive property of the microcapsules was evaluated by an *in vitro* adhesion testing method known as the in vitro wash-off test. Freshly excised pieces of intestinal mucosa (2×2 cm) from sheep were mounted on to glass slides (3×1 inch) with cyanoacrylate glue. Two glass slides were connected with a suitable support. About 50 microspheres were spread on to each wet rinsed tissue specimen and immediately thereafter the support was hanged on to the arm of the USP table disintegrating test machine. When the disintegrating test machine was operated, the tissue specimen was given a slow, regular up-and-down movement in the test fluid at 37°C contained in 1L vessel of the machine. At the end of 1st hr, and at hourly intervals up to 6 hours, the machine was stopped and the number of microspheres still adhering to the tissue was counted. The test was performed in both gastric pH (0.1N HCl, pH 1.2) and intestinal pH (phosphate buffer, pH 7.4).

The optimized gliclazide photomicrograph was showed in Figure 25. The formulated microcapsules were evaluated for various micromeretic properties like bulk density, tapped density, carr's index and hausner's ratio. The results are shown in Table 19. The microcapsules showed good flow properties as they are having carr's index 7.647 and hausner's ratio 1.076. The percentage moisture content and percent loss on drying were also studied and results are mentioned in table 19. The results indicated that the microcapsules had lower % of loss on drying (8.662), which indicated that the microcapsules are free from hygroscopic nature. The wall thickness of the microcapsules was measured and noted as 157.14 μm. The microcapsules also subjected for swelling and erosion studies in phosphate buffer pH-7.4 and results are showed in Figure 26. The results indicated that the % swelling and erosion of the drug from the microcapsules were dependent on time. The extent of swelling was more up to 2.5 hr and then it was decreased. The microcapsules were also subjected to adhesive strength determination by employing in vitro wash off test. This test was conducted in 0.1N HCl and phosphate buffer pH-7.4. The data represented

63

in Figure 27. Results showed higher mucoadhesive strength in 0.1N HCl compared to phosphate buffer pH-7.4.

Figure 25: Photomicrograph of optimized gliclazide microcapsules

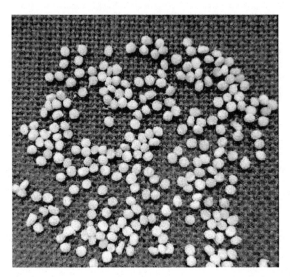

Table 19: Characterization of the optimized gliclazide microcapsules

Parameter	Result
Bulk density (g/ml)	0.693
Tapped density (g/ml)	0.746
Carr's index (%)	7.647
Hausner's ratio	1.076
Wall thickness (μm)	157.14
Moisture content (%)	9.484
Loss on drying (%)	8.662

Figure 26: Percentage swelling and erosion of optimized gliclazide microcapsules in phosphate buffer pH-7.4

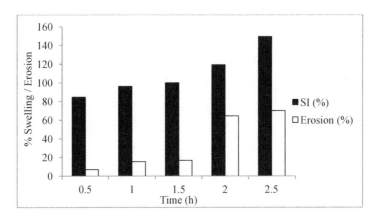

Figure 27: In vitro wash off test data of optimized gliclazide mucoadhesive microcapsules in 0.1N HCl and Phosphate buffer pH-7.4

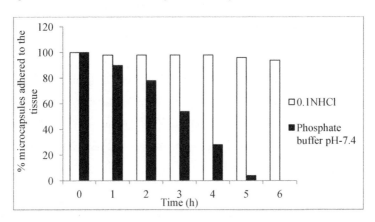

Pharmaco-dynamic studies on rabbits:

Adult albino rabbits weighing between 1.3-1.5kg obtained from the animal house of Bapatla College of pharmacy (1032/ac/07/CPCSEA); Bapatla, were maintained at a constant temperature at $26\pm2°C$, 30-40% RH with 12h light/ dark cycle, throughout the study. The rabbits were housed in clean rabbit cages kept in an air conditioned animal house and were fed with commercial rabbit feed and sterile water. The experimental protocol (IAEC/III/02/BCOP/2011) was approved by the institutional animal ethical committee (IAEC) of Bapatla College of Pharmacy; Bapatla and was in accordance with the guidelines of the committee for the purpose of control and supervision of experimentation of animals.

To study the hypoglycemic activity of gliclazide and its microcapsules, adult healthy albino rabbits were used (n=5). All the animals were fasted for a period of 18 hrs prior to the experiment and water was fed *ad libitum*. The animal dose of gliclzide and its microcapsules was calculated relevant to the human dose (1.4mg/ kg). The required quantity of gliclazide was weighed accurately, dispersed in water. Then the dispersion containing gliclazide equivalent to 1.4mg/kg was administered to the animals orally. The blood samples were collected from the marginal ear vein at 0, 1,2,3,4,6,8,10,12 and 16 hours of post administration. The blood glucose levels were measured using accucheck glucometer. The animals were allowed for one week wash out period. Then the animals were fed with the capsule containing microcapsules equivalent to 1.4mg/kg. The blood samples were collected at the same regular intervals of time and analyzed for the glucose level.

The percent reduction in blood glucose levels was calculated using the following formulae:

$$\% \text{ reduction in blood glucose} = \frac{G0 - Gt}{G0} \times 100$$

G0-Blood glucose concentration at 0th time

Gt- Blood glucose concentration at time (t)

From the blood glucose levels, the percent reduction in blood glucose levels were calculated and shown in Figure 28. The maximum percent reduction of blood glucose was observed at 3rd hour and it was sustained up to 6th hr for pure drug and, however in case of formulation the same effect was observed at 4th hour and extended up to 10th hour. The % reduction in blood glucose levels observed at 3rd and 12th hour were subjected to t-test and very significant differences ($p<0.0001$) were noticed. To compare the variances the data was further subjected to F- test and the result indicated that the differences in variances are not significant ($p=0.6$). This statistical analysis demonstrated that the observed differences in blood glucose levels are due to the differences in mean blood glucose levels (t-test) attributed by the gliclazide and its microcapsules and it also confirmed that the differences in blood glucose levels observed from animal to animal is not significant (variance test).Thus this study clearly indicated that the microcapsules of gliclazide are more effective compared to gliclazide for reduction of blood glucose levels and they can be recommended for once a day administration.

Figure 28: Comparative blood glucose reduction profiles observed from pure drug and microcapsules of gliclazide.

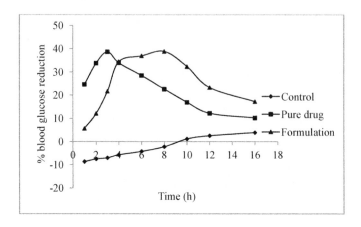

The invitro drug release studies of the optimized gliclazide microcapsules were also conducted in different dissolution mediums such as 0.1N HCl (pH-1.2), acetate buffer (pH-4.5), distilled water (pH-7.0) and phosphate buffer (pH-7.4). The release profiles of optimized formulation were compared (figure 29-31) with the marketed formulation (Azukon MR),similarity factor (f_2) was calculated using the following formulae and the in vitro drug release kinetics showed in Table 20.

$$f_2 = 50 \log \{[1 + \frac{1}{n}\sum_{t=1}^{n}(R_t - T_t)^2)^{-0.5}] \times 100\}$$

These drug release profiles showed good similarity in 0.1N HCl (pH-1.2), acetate buffer (pH-4.5) and phosphate buffer (pH-7.4) and the observed similarity factor (f_2) values were found to be 58.14, 56.62 and 54.53 respectively.

Figure 29: Comparative in vitro drug release profiles of optimized gliclazide microcapsules and gliclazide marketed MR tablet (Azukon) in 0.1N HCl (pH-1.2)

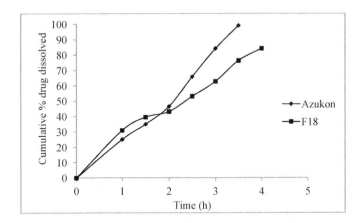

Figure 30: Comparative in vitro drug release profiles of optimized gliclazide microcapsules and gliclazide marketed MR tablet (Azukon) in Acetate buffer (pH-4.5)

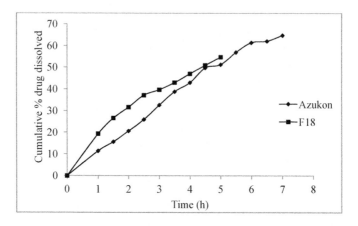

Figure 31: Comparative in vitro drug release profiles of optimized gliclazide microcapsules and gliclazide marketed MR tablet (Azukon) in Phosphate buffer (pH-7.4)

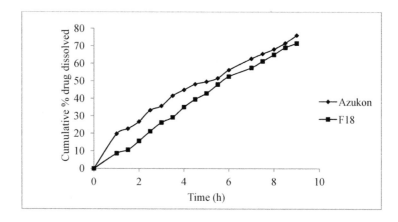

Table 20: In vitro drug release kinetics of optimized gliclazide microcapsules and gliclazide marketed MR tablet (Azukon) in various dissolution media

Dissolution medium employed	Formulation	Correlation coefficient				Release kinetics			Exponential coefficient (n)	Similarity factor (f_2)
		Zero order	First order	Higuchi	Peppas	K mg/h	T_{50} (h)	T_{90} (h)		
0.1N HCl (pH-1.2)	Azukon	0.9913	0.7740	0.9089	0.9788	8.0971	1.9	3.3	0.9121	58.14
	F_{18}	0.9851	0.9552	0.9660	0.9828	6.523	2.3	4.1	0.7245	
Acetate buffer (pH-4.5)	Azukon	0.9918	0.9933	0.9450	0.9916	4.431	4.7	15.6	0.8571	56.62
	F_{18}	0.9399	0.9860	0.9934	0.9970	4.938	4.2	14.0	0.6222	
Phosphate buffer (pH-7.4)	Azukon	0.9586	0.7749	0.9751	0.9866	2.5902	5.8	10.4	0.5942	54.53
	F_{18}	0.9645	0.8641	0.8670	0.9544	2.4836	6.4	11.5	0.7605	

SUMMARY, CONCLUSION AND RECOMMENDATIONS

Studies have been carried out on mucoadhesive microcapsules with an objective of developing microspheres for oral controlled release of gliclazide. Studies were carried out on influence of process variables on encapsulation efficiency and drug release rate. The microspheres were evaluated for micromeritic properties, moisture content, particle size, drug loading, entrapment efficiency, in vitro drug release studies, swelling index, erosion studies, wall thickness and in vitro wash off test. The composition of the optimized formulation was found to be 0.6%w/v sodium alginate, 0.3%w/v of gliclazide and 150ml of 0.1M calcium chloride as curing reagent. The required conditions for the production of microcapsules were found to be an initial stirring of 400 rpm for 60 minutes and allowing for 48hr curing time. The optimized microcapsules provided the slow and controlled drug release up to 12 hrs. The optimized formulation was also subjected to pharmaco-dynamic studies on adult rabbits.

The following **conclusions** were drawn from the present investigation:

1. Gliclazide was found to be compatible with sodium alginate.

2. The encapsulation efficiency and drug release rate from the microcapsules was found to be influenced by the curing time and 48 hr curing time was selected as optimum curing time based on entrapment efficiency and drug release rate.

3. The encapsulation efficiency and drug release rate from the microcapsules was affected by agitation rate and 400 rpm was selected as optimum stirring rate.

4. The drug release was also influenced by stirring time and 60 minutes was found to be optimum stirring time for better drug release.

5. The encapsulation efficiency and drug release rate was affected by volume of curing reagent and 150 ml was selected to be optimum.

6. The encapsulation efficiency and drug release rate was influenced by concentration of curing reagent and 0.1M was found to be optimum.

7. Gliclazide mucoadhesive microcapsules prepared by ionic gelation technique were found to be satisfactory.

8. The drug release from the microcapsules followed zero order kinetics and controlled by non-fickian diffusion mechanism.

9. The microcapsules were found to be spherical and free flowing

10. The prepared microcapsules exhibited good flow properties.

11. The microcapsules showed good swelling properties.

12. The microcapsules exhibited higher mucoadhesive strength in 0.1N HCl compared to phosphate buffer pH-7.4.

13. The microcapsules developed in this investigation showed good similarity with the marketed formulation.

14. The mucoadhesive microcapsules of gliclazide were found to be more suitable in sustaining the hypoglycemic activity compared to gliclazide.

Thus objectives of the present investigation are fulfilled and the results are appropriately discussed.

The following **recommendations** were made for future extension of this research work:

1. Development of suitable pharmaceutically acceptable dosage forms such as tablets, capsules.

2. Identification of suitable storage conditions for preserving the formulation.

3. Selection of suitable packing materials

4. Transfer of this technology to scale up technique

5. Determination of shelf life of the finished dosage form

6. Pharmacokinetic and pharmaco-dynamic studies in animals and human beings

ABBREVIATIONS

mg	milligram
ml	milliliter
μg	microgram
nm	nanometer
cm	centimeter
μm	micrometer
gm	grams
kg	kilograms
min	minutes
h/ hr	hours
rpm	rotations per minute
N	Normality
$\overline{X}$	Mean
S.D.	Standard deviation
n	number of trials
UV	Ultraviolet
IR	Infrared

REFERENCES:

1. Chein, Y.w. rate control drug delivery systems: controlled vs. sustained release, Med. Prog. Techn. 1989, 15, 21-46.

2. Janez Kerc, Three-Phase Pharmaceutical Form ; Three form—with Controlled Release of Amorphous Active Ingredient for Once-Daily Administration2003 Marcel Dekker, Inc. Lek Pharmaceutical and Chemical Company, Ljubljana, Slovenia

3. Ho-wah hui and Joseph Robinson, design and fabrication of oral controlled release drug delivery systems, Marcel Dekker Inc, New york, 1995, 373-378.

4. P.Venkatesan, R.Manavalan and K.Valliappan, Journal of. Pharmaceutical Science & Research, 1 (4), 2009, 26-35.

5. Leon Lachman, Herbert A Liberman, Joseph L. Kanig, The Theory and Practice of Industrial Pharmacy, 3rd edition, Varghese Publishing House, Bombay, 1991,412 .

6. Mathiowitz. E, Jacob. J. S., Jong. Y.S., Carnio. G.P., Chickering. D.E., Chaturvedi. P, Santos. C.A, Vijayaraghavan. K, Monotogomery. S, Basserr. M and Morrell. C, Nature, 1997, 386 (6623), 410-414.

7. K. P. R. Chowdary and Y. Srinivasa Rao, Biol. Pharma. Bull. 2004; 27(11); 1717-1724.

8. Mathiowitz, Donald E. Chickering III, Bioadhesive Drug Delivery Systems, Fundamental Novel Approaches & Development, Marcel Dekker, Inc, Newyork, 1999, 1-5.

9. G.P. Andrews et al., Eur. J. Pharm. Biopharm, 2009, 71, 505-518.

10.Gandhi R.B., Robinson J.R., Ind. J. Pharm. Sci., 1988, 50(3), 145-152.

11.Chen J.L., Cyr. G.N., Composition producing adhesion through hydration. In mainly R.S., ed., Adhesion in biological system. New York; Academic Press, 163-181.

12.Roy, K. Pal, A. Anis, K. Pramanik and B.Prabhakar, Designed monomers and polymers 12 (2009), 483-495.

13.Allur, H.H., Johnston, T.P. and Mitra, A.K., In; Swarbrick,J. and Boylan, J.C., Eds., Encyclopedia of Pharmaceutical Technology, 1990,20(3) , Marcel Dekker, New York, 193-218.

14.Y. Huang, W. Leobandung, A. Foss, N.A. Peppas, J. Control. Release 65, 2000, 63-71.

15.Y. Sudhakar, K. Kuotsu, A.K. Bandyopadhyay, J. Control. Release 114, 2006, 15-40.

16.H. Sigurdsson, T. Loftsson, C. Lehr, Int. J. Pharm. 325, 2006, 75-81.

17.E. A. Kharenko, N. I. Larionova, and N. B. Demina, Mucoadhesive Drug Delivery Systems (Review), Translated from Khimiko-Farmatsevticheskii Zhurnal, 43 (4), 2009, 21 – 29.

18.Ch'ng H.S., Park H., Kelly P., Robinson J.R.J. Pharm. Sci, 1985, 74,399-405

19.Pranshu Tangri, International Journal of Pharma Research and Development – Online, ISSN 0974 – 9446, Publication Ref No.:

IJPRD/2011/PUB/ARTI/VOV-3/ISSUE-2/APRIL/018 accessed on 10-6-2011.

20. Vasir. J.K., Tambwekar. K and Garg. S, Int. J. Pharmaceutics, 2003, 255 (1-2), 13-32

21. Edith Mathiowitz, Encyclopedia of controlled Drug Delivery, Bioadhesive drug delivery systems, A Wiley-Interscience Publication, John Wiley & Sons, Inc., New York, volume I, 14-17.

22. Botagataj, M., Mrhar, A. and Korosec, L., Int. J. Pharm., 177, 1999, 211-20

23. Sam AP, Van Dan Heuij JT, Tukker J. Int J Pharm, 53, 1989, 97-105

24. D. Fei, Determination of gliclazide in tablets by UV spectrophotometry, Yaowu- aFenxi- Zazhi, 1992, 12, 116–117.

25. S.A. Hussein, A.M.I. Mohamed, A.A.M. Abdel-Alim, Utility of certain pi-acceptors for the spectrophotometric determination of gliclazide and tolazamide, Analyst, 1989, 114, 1129–1131.

26. T. Maeda, T.Yamaguchi, M. Hashimoto, Gas-chromatographic determination of the hypoglycaemic agent gliclazide in plasma, J. Chromatogr.Biomed, 1981, 12, 357–363.

27. M. Kimura, K. Kobayashi, M. Hata, S. Takashima, T. Ino, A. Matsuoka,et al., Determination of gliclazide in human plasma by highperformance liquid chromatography and gas chromatography, Hyogo-Ika- Daigaku-Igakkai-Zasshi,1980, 5, 49–55.

28. N.M. El-Kousy, Stability-indicating densitometric determination of some antidiabetic drugs in dosage forms, using TLC, Mikrochim. Acta, 1998, 128, 65–68.

29. D. Zhang, J.Z. Zeng, Y. Jiang, J.D. Chao, T. Li, Determination and pharmacokinetic study of gliclazide in human plasma by HPLC, Yaowu- Fenxi- Zazhi, 1996, 16, 157–159.

30. Y.Q. Hu, H.C. Liu, X.F. Li, G.W. Zhu, Analysis of gliclazide in human serum by high-performance liquid chromatography (HPLC), Sepu, 1995, 13, 227–228.

31. R. Nadkarni–Deepali, R.N. Merchant, M. Sundaresan, A.M. Bhagwat, Isocratic separation and simultaneous estimation of four antidiabetic members of the sulphonyl urea family by reversed-phase HPLC, Indian Drugs, 1997, 34,650–653.

32. Y. Wang, Y.J. Wang, Z.P. Liu, L.B. Yu, Y.P.F.H. Shi, et al., HPLC determination of gliclazide in human plasma by reversed-phase high performance liquid chromatography, Sepu, 1993, 11, 352–354.

33. British Pharmacopeia, vol. I and II, Her Majesty's Stationary Office, London, 1998, 637–638.

34. H. Kajinuma, K. Ichikawa, Y. Akanuma, K. Kosaka, N. Kuzuya, Radio-immunoassay for gliclazide in serum.I. Validity of the assay, and change in serum level after intra-venous administration, Tonyobyo, 1982, 25, 869–875.

35. Raida S. Al-Kassas, Omaimah M.N. Al-Gohary, Monirah M. Al-Faadhel, International Journal of Pharmaceutics, 2007, 341, 230–237.

36. Shabaraya AR, Narayanacharyulu R, Indian journal of pharmaceutical sciences, 2003, 65 (3), 250-252.

37. Zinutti, C and Hoffman M, J. Microencao., 11 (5), 1994, 555-563.

38. Sustained-release formulation of gliclazide, European patent application, EP 2 181 705 A1

39. Parul Trivedi, A M L Verma, N Garud, Asian journal of pharmaceutics, 2008, 110-115.

40. Leon Lachman, Herbert A Liberman, Joseph L. Kanig, The Theory and Practice of Industrial Pharmacy, 3rd edition, Varghese Publishing House, Bombay, 1991, 52.

41. Desai KG, Park HJ, Drug delivery, 2006, 13, 39-50

42. Si-Nang, L, Carlier, P.F., Delort, p, Gazzola, J and Labont, D, J. Pharm. Sci., 1973, 62 (3), 452-455.

43. Lehr, C.M., Bowstra, J.A., Tukker, J.J. and Junginer, H.E., J. Control. Rel., 1990, 13 (1), 51-62.

44. K.P.R.Chowdary and Y. Srinivasa Rao, Indian journal of pharmaceutical sciences, 2003, 65 (3), 279-284.

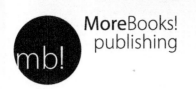
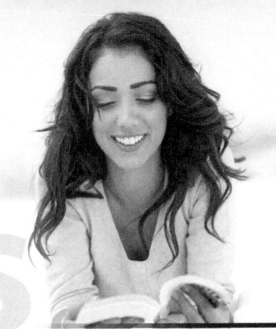

Printed in Great Britain
by Amazon

25429172R00050